REBOUNDING AND YOUR IMMUNE SYSTEM

Optimal Support For Your Body's Natural Defense

By
Linda Brooks
Certified Reboundologist

Vitally Yours Press
Eaton, Ohio

Printed in the United States of America

Second Printing November, 2004

Rebounding and Your Immune System

By
Linda Brooks
Certified Reboundologist

Please write or call me for more information on:

Rebounders, stabilizer bars, books, and videos
Personal rebound exercise programs
Certified Reboundologist workshops
Seminars and speaking engagements
Vital Health News bi-monthly newsletter
(Look for order information at the end of this book.)

Linda Brooks
Vitally Yours

109 Revere Dr, Greensboro, NC 27407
877-299-9547 336-547-8191
reboundvy@aol.com www.2rebound.com

www.2rebound.com

I dedicate this book to my "rebound-loving" mother, Margaret Brooks, who believed in me and the work that I do to teach others about its awesome benefits.

Disclaimer

The information in this book is not intended to be a substitute for medical advice in any case. The author is offering information only, which is not medical advice or a remedy for any medical condition.

About Your Author

Linda Brooks has had experience with rebound exercise since 1980. She became a Certified Reboundologist in 1991 and did graduate study in nutrition at UNCG in North Carolina.

Her Vitally Yours program allows the body to heal itself by providing the simplest, most basic, natural needs of the cells. Linda has been a distributor of the NEEDAK rebounder since 1991.

Linda teaches others to be Certified Reboundologists with her CR workshop that she teaches around the country on demand. This is a very experiential workshop covering all aspects of therapeutic and aerobic rebounding.

Linda enjoys researching, writing other publications, and producing educational videos on rebounding, which she calls the "ultimate exercise."

"Rebounding is a most satisfying way of life for me. It exemplifies simplicity, efficiency, economy and good health. I think of it as a fountain of youth."

Other publications by Linda:

Rebounding To Better Health
Cancer — A Simple Approach
***Vital Health News* newsletter**
***Bounce Before You Jump* video**
***What Comes After The Bounce* video**
***A Beginner's Workout* video**

Vitally Yours
Mission Statement

The Vitally Yours Center For Cellular Health program is designed to help people achieve vibrant health through education and the use of basic tools that meet the needs of the body on a cellular level, resulting in the body being able to heal itself as it naturally knows how to do.

This simple, very basic approach of internal cleansing, optimal nutrition, ideal exercise through rebounding, and emotional and spiritual awareness lets the body reach homeostasis without the use of traditional invasive techniques.

The Vitally Yours program respects the individuality of the healing process. Each person begins at their level of awareness and proceeds at his or her own pace. Some may start with nutrition, some with rebounding, some with emotional issues, while others begin spiritually.

One level of healing leads to another, as the individual accepts the basic truths about the ability to heal in body, mind, and spirit. The body is the miracle, seeking, and maintaining balance as its basic, cellular needs are met.

~~~Linda Brooks

This program, is not presented as medical advice, in any case, nor are any of the products suggested in this program intended as medical use or prescription. This program contains information and suggested products designed for educational purposes only.
~~~

Thank You!

Because the readers of my first book and also many clients wanted more information on the body's defense system, I decided to write it down simply in a short, yellow booklet in the year 2000, called *Rebounding and Your Lymphatic System.* That short booklet was very popular and I printed quick copies on demand for over two years.

That "little yellow book," as it was often called, has been expanded to fit the format of my other two books in my series of educational books on rebounding. The cover remains yellow, however, it is now titled *Rebounding and Your Immune System,* and contains more information on your body's natural defense, plus exciting stories from others who want to share their successful experiences of rebounding.

My thanks go to those of you who have waited patiently for the update and expansion of this "little yellow book." Your interest and need have kept the wheels of progress, slow as it has been at times, steadfastly turning.

Thanks to NEEDAK Manufacturing, and those dealers who support my writings by sharing my books with their clients.

Proofreading seems to never end. Big thanks go to Kay and Judy for helping me make it make sense to my readers.

Many thanks go to all the individual people who are intrigued and in love with rebounding and just soak up truth when presented clearly to them, then come back looking for more.

Introduction

This is the third in a series of educational books conveying basic truths about how rebound exercise meets the needs of your body, cell by cell. Rebounding is a balancing experience that turns on the body's ability to heal itself.

For this I am truly grateful, because 20 years ago I was too sick to write this book, and many times prior to that, to truly enjoy my life and be effective in what I was doing.

From a liver infection at the age of six, to antibiotics, to ear infections, colds, flu, pneumonia, more antibiotics, hormone imbalance, low blood sugar, and exhaustion, to overweight and being tired of being tired, I wanted to feel better, but not with more drugs and pills.

I started searching for answers about how my body worked, and what it needed to work efficiently. After making some dietary changes, rebound exercise found me in 1980, and I got excited! I had been jogging to gain some energy and lose some weight.

Working up to jogging three miles a day helped me feel better, but after a while I didn't like the pressure I was beginning to feel in my knees and ankles. When I entered the House of Health in Greensboro, North Carolina in early September of 1980, I had no idea that my life was about to change. Rand Pack, owner of the store who usually watched me select vitamins and minerals of all kinds, took me to the back of the store to show me a rebounder. I got on and bounced with joy and then discovered I could run on it without discomfort at all!

Oh, happy day! Rand gave me a little book by Al Carter that I read from cover to cover several times. I bounced and jumped and ran on that magical device and my body started to respond with better health. Everything got better.

The greatest benefit from all my easy, fun bounces was getting my immune system up to par again. Less sinus infections, less ear infections, less allergies, and as time went on, no more sinus, ear, or allergy problems. Rebounding helped clean out and clean up my system from old and damaged cells, toxins, stored residues of medications, and who knows what else!

It didn't happen over night, since my body had been through medications, damaged cells, and mental stresses. I learned that changing to a natural, and later, vegetarian diet also helped my body rebuild more efficiently. I was on a role.

My immune system has responded so favorably that I can honestly say that I rarely have anything significant bother me. It's great to go through entire winters without pneumonia and ear infections, and to be able to mow grass in the summer without my sinuses getting messed up. None of that has happened for years!

When I was getting low blood sugar under control years ago, a naturally oriented doctor told me he believed the future of our health lay in the realm of immunology. With what I knew then about the physiology of the human body from my graduate study in nutrition, I knew he was on to something. That outstanding concept has remained with me and has been proven to be true, as I see the results of immune support in myself and others, over and over again.

There is a myriad of immune system boosters available in the way of herbs, nutritional formulas, and body work techniques, however, rebound exercise stands out above them all.

I will explain its powerful lymphatic flushing and benefits to all cells that no other exercise can give, but first, let's find out what this vaguely known immune system is all about.

Table of Contents

"The voyage of discovery lies not in finding new landscapes, but in having new eyes."

~~~Marcel Proust
~~~

Chapter One

Your Immune System

Your immune system is probably the least understood system in the human body, and yet, it is your body's number one line of defense. Your immune system is designed to keep you healthy, no matter what. It can defend you against cancer and help you heal from anything from serious illness to the common cold.

Where have you learned about your immune system functions in the past? Surely in general health classes in junior high school, you learned a little about how lymph carries garbage away, and about how white blood cells work as soldiers of defense. But what about how it really works on the cellular level, and its potential to heal you **no matter what?**

Just what can you expect from your immune system? If it is your defense system, then why do you get sick? What causes the breakdowns, followed by getting well again? Your body has an innate intelligence for healing that goes beyond your wildest imagination.

We have grown accustomed to the many band aids that the medical profession offers from the drug giants. We also are weary that we haven't found satisfactory answers with them. Now as we peel off the layers of unsuccessful approaches that cover the vibrant health we know is possible, it is time to pull back and know the simple truths involved with wellness, get out of our own way, and let the body heal itself.

The information in this book is basic. There are no band aid approaches needed when you stimulate your body's defense system and meet the basic needs of the cells, physically, emotionally, and spiritually.

The human body is a miracle. Viruses? Cancer? Colds? Flu? MS? Chronic Fatigue? Diabetes? Arthritis? Allergies? Lupus? Edema? Tonsillitis? Measles? Lyme Disease? Fibromyalgia? Lethargy? Headaches? Foggy Thinking? Depression? Pain? Have you limited your expectations of healing from some of these and other illnesses? What happens to block the defense system and allow illness to prevail?

Circumstances and events around you everyday have a profound effect on your immune system. Diet, exercise, stress level, beliefs, spiritual growth, and other factors effect your level of defense from day to day.

My Vitally Yours basic program for health describes how to meet the body's needs on the cellular level so you can achieve optimal defense and healing from your body, based on it's own natural intelligence.

Learning to expect your body to heal itself, once its basic needs are met, may bring about some changes in your beliefs about your body and the potential of its intelligence.

Let's look at this fascinating system of defense and what is necessary to keep it operating at an optimal level of performance, while you are dealing with environmental toxins, computer and office strain, fatigue, emotional stresses, and a myriad of other circumstances that may lower your level of defense.

My approach is to work on the cellular level and to make sure the cells are receiving what they need, including proper housecleaning and defense against invaders. All the systems of the body work together to support the health of the whole, likewise, a breakdown in one area affects the health of the entire body in some way.

The Basic Set Up

Your miraculous immune system is your body's number one line of defense, holistically created to help you stay well and get well, should you become ill, in spite of many factors that affect its efficiency.

Your immune system is composed of:

Lymphatic vessels — These are lymph veins and lymph capillaries that run throughout the body, usually running parallel to arteries and veins, and used for the transport of cellular debris. This is a closed system, not directly connected to the blood circulatory system. Sixty percent are in the skin.

Lymphatic organs — Lymph nodes, thymus gland, spleen, adenoids, and appendix are in this group.

White blood cells — Neutraphils, eosinophils, basophils, lymphocytes, monocytes, natural killer cells, etc. These cells are very structured and orderly.

Specialized cells — macrophages and mast cells.

Specialized chemical fractions — Interferon, interleukins, and complement fractions produced in the liver and spleen.

Skin — Largest defense organ in the body. It secretes antibacterial substances.

Tears and mucus — Break down the cell wall of many bacteria with their lysozyme enzyme.

Colds, flu, infections, and serious illness such as cancer, only occur when the immune system is weakened or compromised in some way. Keeping this system operating optimally is of prime importance to your health.

Your Lymphatic System

We tend to think of our lymphatic system as our waste removal, or garbage system, for the bloodstream and the cells. It is truly that, and more. It is of utmost importance that this system operate efficiently, for if it were to shut down for 24 hours, the human body could not survive.

Briefly, the lymphatic functions are:

1. Flow of lymph along lymphatic veins.
2. Return of blood proteins to circulation.
3. Filtration of the lymph by the lymph nodes.

Approximately one-sixth of the body is space between the cells, which is filled with lymph, also called extra-cellular fluid, or interstitial fluid, that surrounds or bathes each cell. Lymph is also found flowing through a series of tubes called lymphatic veins. Healthy lymph is clear and flows through the lymphatic vessels freely. There is three to four times as much lymph as blood in the body, yet because the lymph has no physical pump, it flows very slowly, depending on constant movement of some kind in the body for its flow through the body toward the heart.

The millions of lymphatic terminals at the ends of the lymphatic veins are attached to the surrounding tissues by little hair-like strings called ***anchoring filaments.*** When a tissue fills with excess fluid around the cells, the anchoring filaments wiggle, opening the doors to the lymphatic veins.

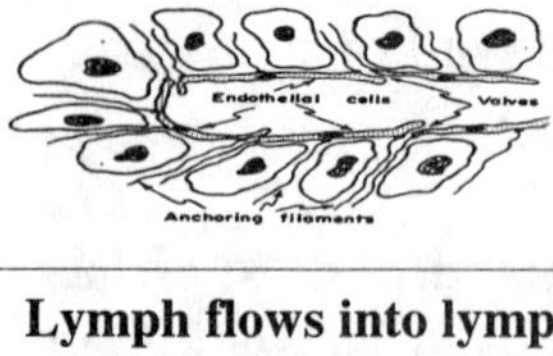

Lymph flows into lymph vein when body movement causes anchoring filaments to open doorway into vein.

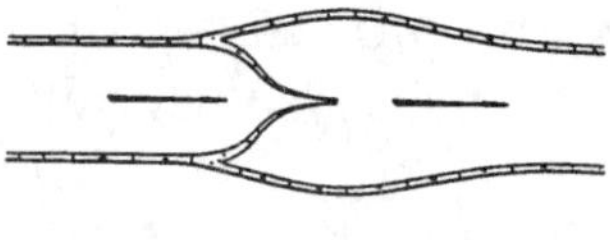

Lymph moves through a series of one-way valves in lymphatic veins, to reach subclavian vein.

The lymph fluid flows into the veins, or lymphatic chambers. It cannot backwash because the cells lining the vessels overlap each other, opening in, and acting as one-way doors that allow the fluid to flow only one way. One-way valves inside the lymph veins keep the lymph from pooling in the feet!

The lymph fluid flows through this series of thin veins with one-way valves oriented so that the lymph continuously flows toward the subclavian vein, near the heart, where it empties back into circulation. It never flows backward toward the tissues.

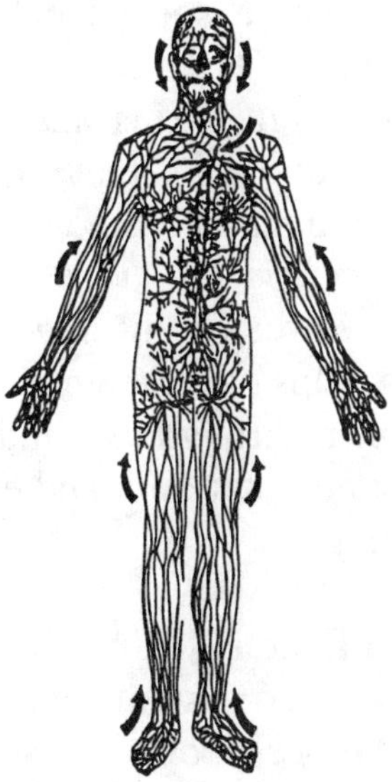

Direction of Lymphatic Drainage

The lymph flows through this system of one-way valves toward the heart like a hydraulic pressure system. When the pressure below a valve is greater than that above the valve, the fluid flows up, causing the valve to open. The lymph fluid gets pumped by movement from your toes up through the lymph nodes positioned near your joints and throughout your body, to the heart.

Tiny muscles around the lymph capillary that are sensitive to the pressure of the lymph-filled vessel contract and force the fluid on to the next chamber. Additional pumping can be caused by movement and bending of the arms and legs, and by breathing. Any movement around the lymph vessels as well as arterial pulsations, can help squeeze the fluid toward the heart, where it empties into the subclavian vein, to be further cleansed by the liver and kidneys.

Continuous flow of lymphatic fluid means continuous cleansing of the cells. Lack of regular exercise and physical movement means stagnation of lymph and can lead to poisoning of the cells.

As the lymph flows along its pathway through the one-way valves, it passes through hundreds of filters, called lymph nodes, where special cells attack and digest foreign protein molecules. Other cells form antibodies to protect the system from foreign toxins and bacteria. In these recycling centers, many amino acids that come from protein molecules are designated to be used by the body.

Forceful flushing of the lymph fluid through the lymph nodes helps clean the nodes. It is like squirting a forceful spray of water through a window screen rather than dropping a trickle of water on it and expecting the screen to be cleaned effectively.

Exercise moves lymph. Your body is made for movement — consistent movement. **Non-exercisers are seven times more prone to be affected by degenerative diseases such as heart problems, cancer, arthritis, and diabetes than those who exercise regularly.** Regular rebound exercise, because of its increased pull of gravity, is the most efficient exercise for moving lymph.

Lethargy, foggy thinking, depression, headaches, and anxiety could be signs of an inefficient immune system, where toxins accumulate in the body, interfering with normal body functions.

The spinal fluid, bathing the brain and spine, is part of the lymphatic system. Some 57 different chemicals are secreted in this fluid, therefore, exercise affects our emotions and nervous system in a positive way.

Rebound exercise cleanses all cells and balances the production of brain chemicals.

The Problem With Edema

A common condition resulting from a break down in efficient lymphatic flow is the swelling of certain body areas, most often the lower extremities, called edema. Extra lymph is held between the cells causing pressure, pain, infection, and in extreme cases, gangrene. This is a very troublesome condition for many individuals and is an indication that the lymphatic system is not functioning efficiently.

Let's look at how the lymph system normally keeps the tissues from holding extra fluid, and what conditions may exist if lymphatic flow is inhibited.

Because of the normal pressure of the blood flow throughout the body, there is a small rate of leakage of blood proteins from the plasma. This is because some of the capillary pores are just the right size for some of the blood proteins to get squeezed through to the outside of the capillary by the beating of the heart. Now they are in the lymph between cells where there is not enough pressure to return them to the bloodstream. Each hour, 1/25 of the total proteins in circulation is squeezed out of the capillaries.

This activity is a natural occurrence in the human body and does not signify anything wrong. The only danger lies in the immune system being compromised so that the blood proteins become trapped and are not promptly returned to circulation.

These blood proteins normally get promptly returned to circulation by way of the lymphatic system. The blood proteins sitting in the lymph between the cells enter the lymphatic veins and are pumped by movement through the one-way valve chambers to the subclavian vein where they go back into circulation.

If these proteins were never returned to the bloodstream, death would occur within 12-24 hours because of the negative effects of the edema state.

Proteins pushed outside the blood capillary will attract water around them if they are not returned to circulation by way of the lymphatic system. The extra fluid pushes the cells away from the capillary, causing swelling, or edema. These blood proteins become trapped, because normal flow of lymph has been compromised. This impairs the transport of nutrients and oxygen to the cells, sometimes so seriously that some of the cells die. When the lymphatic flow is impaired, the dead cells, being trapped, can putrefy and send toxins through the

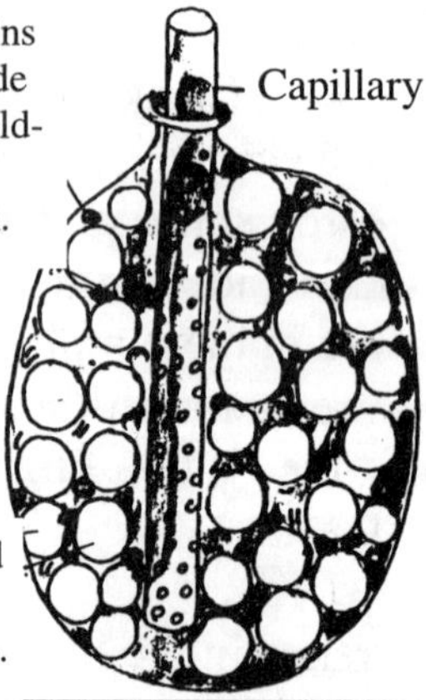

Unhealthy edema state

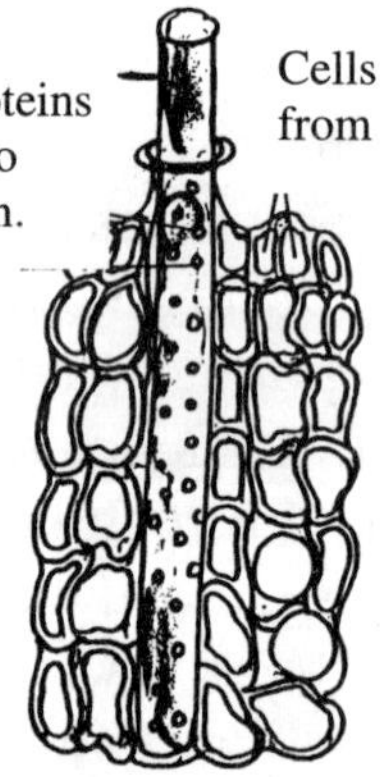

Healthy "dry" state

"The return of proteins to circulation is the single most important function of the lymphatic system." (Arthur C. Guyton, author of *Functions of The Human Body*, and authority on the lymphatic system.)

system.

Common causes of edema are injury, lack of exercise, sluggish lymph, and clogged lymph nodes. When these trapped blood proteins attract fluid around them and shut off nutrients and oxygen to the cells, the potential for degenerative disease and illness sets in.

To return these blood proteins to circulation and reduce the edema, it is most important to stimulate the immune system and flush the lymphatic fluid throughout the body.

Rebound exercise stimulates the forceful flow of all the lymph fluid so the extra fluid in the edema area is pumped away from the cells and the blood proteins that are stuck in the lymph are returned to circulation.

Tissue cells then return to their healthy position of lying close to each other and close to the blood capillaries where they can receive food and oxygen efficiently. Swelling is eliminated, and with continued rebound exercise, the ***cause*** of the swelling is also eliminated.

Strengthening of all the cells is experienced so injuries can heal, sluggish, milky lymph becomes clear and able to flow freely again, and the congestion in the lymph nodes is cleared out with the forceful flow of lymph.

Your body's defense system has ideal support with rebound exercise, and it only takes two minutes of health bouncing repeated several times a day to achieve it.

Health bouncing for two minutes every hour, or at least 5-6 times a day relieves edema and its cause and gives better support to your immune system than one long rebound session.

In extreme cases of edema, buddy bounces (see page 32)

may be employed comfortably. In any case, be creative and bounce, bounce, bounce!

Rebounding works, and it is important to find a program that meets your body's needs and your enjoyment.

Chapter Two

The Immune System: A Closer Look

Functions of lymphatics:

Removes foreign substances from the blood and lymph
Combats disease
Maintains tissue fluid balance by returning blood proteins to circulation
Absorbs fat

Natural Fighters:

Leucocytes: White blood cells, nucleated, involved in immunity.
Five types of Leucocytes: Neutrophils, eosinophils, basophils, lymphocytes, and monocytes.

Neutrophils: Phagocytic (eating) white blood cells that ingest bacteria. They also ingest tissue debris, clearing the area for tissue repair. Neutrophils are killed in action, and can accumulate as dead cells and fluid, called **pus.**

Over half the army of white blood cells designed to fight disease is made up of neutrophils which are made in the bone marrow. **When called upon, they change shape to fit better through the vessels of the body. On the scene, they stick a tiny foot (pseudopod) through any tiny crack that may exist, and engulf the invader with their own bodies and quickly digest it.** The neutrophils come in waves until the job is done.

Eosinophils: White blood cells involved in **regulating the inflammatory process, releasing chemicals that reduce inflammation.** Chemicals from eosinophils are also involved with the **destruction of worm parasites.**

Basophils: Neucleated white blood cells involved in the inflammatory response. Basophils release histamine and other chemicals that promote inflammation. **Basophils also contain heparin, which prevents the formation of blood clots.**

Lymphocytes: **Smallest of the leucocytes (B and T cells)** with diverse activities that involve the **production of antibodies and other chemicals that destroy pathogens,** contribute to allergic reactions, reject grafts, control tumors, and regulate the immune system. They are called lymphocytes because they are transported through the lymph fluid. Lymphocytes are born in the bone marrow and produce proteins called antibodies found in the plasma.

B cells: The first of the lymphocytes to be discovered. They produce tiny proteins called antibodies that attach to **extracellular** bacteria, viruses and foreign invaders (antigens). Each B lymphocyte produces only one kind of antibody; one attacks the cold, another attacks bacteria in pneumonia, etc. B cells are born and mature in the bone marrow, and circulate in the blood and lymph fluid.

T cells: These lymphocytes are born in the bone marrow, and mature in the thymus gland where they get their training. They get their name, **T** cells, from the word **t**hymus. A small number of them stand alert in the lymph nodes and spleen which have specialized compartments for different kinds of immune system cells. T cells do not produce antibodies, but directly **attack intracellular foreign invaders.** They produce lymphokines, chemicals that activate macrophages and other immune cells; promote phagocytosis and inflammation. There are several kinds of T cells, each having different functions.

Monocytes: Largest of the leucocytes. They may leave the blood and transform to become macrophages which **phagocytize (eat) bacteria, dead neutrophils, cell fragments, and any other debris within the tissues.**

Cytotoxic T cells: Killing cells that attack only one kind of infected cell or agent, such as cancer cells, viruses, etc.

Natural Killer cells (NK): Constantly patrol the body looking for dangerous foreign cells. When they find a dangerous cell they attach to it and release toxic chemicals that destroy the invading cells. NK cells are known to be involved in defense against cancer by scavenging normal cells that go awry.

Helper T cells: Stimulate B lymphocytes to make antibodies. They release a protein called interleuken 2, which stimulates the lymphocytes to divide.

Suppressor T cells: Designed to keep the immune system from getting out of control. They shut off helper T cells once enough antibodies are made.

Other pertinent terms relating to the immune system

Lacteals: Special lymph vessels called lacteals are located in the lining of the small intestine, specifically, inside the villi. Fats enter the lacteals and pass through the lymph veins to the blood. The lymph passing through these lymph vessels has a milky appearance because of its fat content.

Antigens: Substances that cause the immune system to produce antibodies. Antigens can be made within the body, called self antigens, or come from outside, called foreign antigens.

Thymus gland: The main function of the thymus is to **develop immature T cells**. This process begins with the production of pre-T cells in the bone marrow and their subsequent transport to the thymus via the blood. The pre-T cells are then taken into the cortex where a series of molecular events takes place allowing the cells to recognize certain antigens.

Spleen: The largest mass of lymphatic tissue in the body, weighing about 7 ounces. The spleen behaves similar to a lymph node, but instead of filtering the lymphatic fluid, it filters the blood. **It destroys worn out red blood cells, responds to foreign substances in the blood, and is a reservoir for blood.**

Thoracic duct: The **largest lymph vessel in the body**. It drains the left side of the head and neck, the upper thorax, the left upper limb, and the inferior half of the body into the left subclavian vein.

Lymph nodes: Specialized dilations of lymphatic tissue which are supported within by a meshwork of connective tissue called reticulin fibers and are populated by dense aggregates of lymphocytes and macrophages. Lymph nodes appear along the entire length of the lymphatic system and tend to increase in size as they become closer to the thoracic duct. They are also **organized in chains that drain exclusively a particular organ or region of the body**.

Both arteries and veins enter the nodes so their leucocytes can be quickly dumped into the bloodstream. Most lymph nodes are bean shaped and about one inch in length. The node is divided into compartments called trabeculae, but has two basic parts, the cortex and the medulla. The cortex is populated mainly with lymphocytes. B cells rest in the germinal centers and in the event of an infecting antigen, the B cells will rapidly undergo mitosis and divide. This could cause

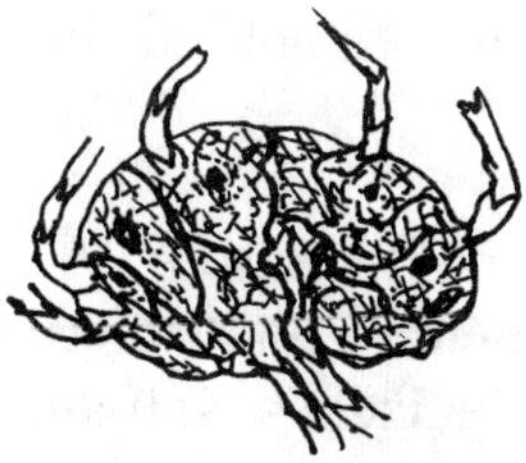

Normal lymph node

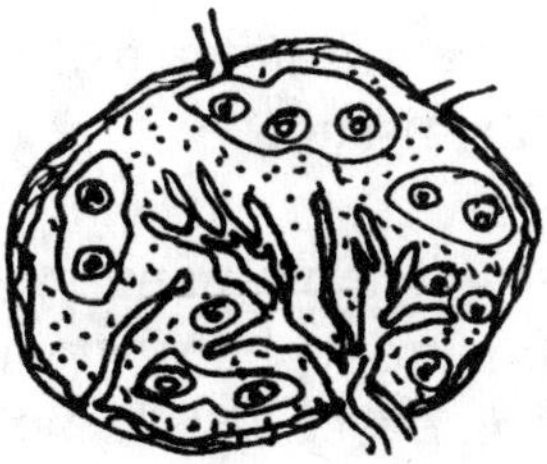

Swollen lymph node

swelling of the lymph node, indicating immune activity.

The rest of the cortex contains T cells that circulate through the lymph nodes, blood stream, and lymphatic ducts. The medulla section of the node primarily contains macrophages attached to reticular fibers.

Interleukin-1: Secreted by the macrophages, this protein **activates T helper cells** and causes the brain to raise the body temperature, which increases the efficiency of the immune system.

Interleukin-2: Secreted by the T helper cells, this protein **signals the production of T killer cells.**

Endorphins: Natural pain killers, known as the natural "opiates" of the brain. Any activity that produces a reported "high" is accompanied by endorphin increase and enhancement of the immune system. They invigorate the attack on cancer by T killer cells and also increase the number, percentage, and effectiveness of the immune cells. **Endorphins are 5-10 times more powerful than morphine.**

Immunoglobulins: Antibodies that have different functions. There are 5 classes (IbG, IgM, IgA, IgE, and IgD) of these globulin proteins.

Autoimmune disease: The immune system treats self antigens as foreign antigens, stimulating unwanted destruction of normal tissue.

The immune system contains receptors for endorphins and neuropeptides traveling throughout the entire body, contacting every cell. If the system does not recognize a cell, it attacks it.

The immune system responds to chemicals and secretes chemical messages.

There are connections between the immune system and the central nervous system. The immune system has nerve cells that connect the brain to the spleen and other organs producing immune cells. Stress has a very negative effect on the immune system, which is explained later in this book.

Communication between the immune cells occurs by way of interferons, interleukens, and other chemical messengers that govern the immune system.

Chapter Three

How Rebound Exercise Works

Rebound exercise strengthens every cell of the body equally at the same time. This is accomplished by the **triple force** placed on each cell on the down bounce. As you bounce, you are accelerating and decelerating on the same plane, or vertically, with gravity. During other exercise such as walking, running, and tennis, your acceleration and deceleration are on the horizontal plane. In normal exercise, you *oppose gravity with just one force.*

In 1911, Albert Einstein showed that when the forces of acceleration and deceleration are aligned in the same plane as gravity, the body feels all three forces as if they are each gravity. The cells of the body know how to adjust to an increased force of gravity. They respond by getting stronger.

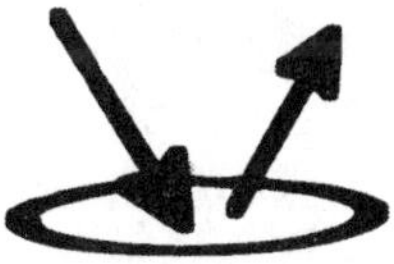

Another way of stating this process is that a **loaded force** is placed on every cell, or on the down bounce the cells are loaded, and they adapt to the load by getting stronger. Rebound exercise is resistance training for each cell. Each cell weighs more at the bottom of the bounce, so it adjusts to the increased gentle force by getting stronger.

In a N.A.S.A. study comparing treadmill running to rebound running, rebound exercise is shown to be 68% more effective to the total body.

Another major benefit to rebound exercise is that it flushes the entire lymphatic system and triples white blood cells in two minutes of health bouncing.

As you bounce up and down, your cells experience a gentle squeezing at the bottom of the bounce, pulling toxins from the cells.The change in gravitational pull at the top of the bounce causes all the one-way valves in the lymph veins to open, allowing lymph to flow freely. At the bottom of the bounce, toxins are forced out of the cells, and as pressure changes on the upward bounce, toxins enter the lymph veins to be pumped to the subclavian vein where they proceed to the liver and kidneys to be further filtered and expelled.

Because lymph is moving and dead white blood cells and toxins are being expelled, *the demand for white blood cells increases.* Two minutes of gentle bouncing stimulates the white blood cell count to approximately triple in number. This army of white blood cells works to kill cancer cells, and clear debris and toxins from the cells for about one hour. After that time, the white blood cell count is back to normal, so **the two minute health bounce can be repeated every hour to keep the immune system operating optimally.**

A stronger, cleaner body can function better and provides the environment for healing to take place. There are as many benefits of rebound exercise as there are processes in the human body, since every single process taking place in the body is enhanced by rebounding.

Rebound exercise provides a forceful flow of lymph along the lymph pathways, that effectively cleanses all the cells and cleans the lymph nodes, or filters, as well.

Many herbs and nutritional supplements have the ability also to enhance the effectiveness of the immune system, however, **rebound exercise goes beyond that enhancement and provides the forceful flushing of all the lymph fluid so all the cells of the body are cleaned at once.**

Rebound exercise also is a valuable tool that provides

the return of blood proteins to circulation, eliminating the cause for edema. As certain blood proteins get squeezed out of the capillaries by the heart beat, they are returned through the lymphatic system to circulation, instead of being trapped.

Rebound Moves

The basic groups of moves, including several aerobic bounces, are illustrated in my book, *Rebounding To Better Health*, and demonstrated on my video, *Bounce Before You Jump.*

The first thing to understand when moving on the rebounder, is that rebounding applies a compact, triple force of gravity to each cell, and that **it is extremely important not to overdo!** Many people believe that if health bouncing is good, fun, and so easy, then it will be helpful to go higher or at a more intense pace. Not everyone is ready for that right away. **Too much too soon can cause weak areas of the body to get sore, so find your starting point and go slowly.**

You can develop a safe, effective, and enjoyable program, whatever your condition. Anyone can rebound.

You do not have to follow a certain routine, or "work" hard in order to receive benefits from rebounding. **It is quite beneficial to just do the health bounce, keeping your feet on the mat, if that is all you want to do, or perhaps is all that you are able to do at this time.** You should work on your own level and proceed gradually. Consistency is an important key to success. Rebounding is an everyday exercise, with no excuses.

1. **Health Bounce:** Gently bounce with your **feet on the mat** and feet about 12 inches apart. Shrug your shoulders or slightly lift your heels to get yourself bouncing. The buoyancy of the springs on a quality rebounder will keep you going with

little of your effort. This bounce strengthens every cell, flushes lymphatics, increases white blood cells, and improves circulation while also enhancing every bodily process, thus the name *health bounce.*

2. **Strength Bounce:** Jump up and down on the mat to increase the G-force on each cell. **The strength bounce is done by actually leaving the mat on the upward bounce.** Those with joint and back weaknesses or other injuries should avoid jumping and do the health bounce, exclusively, until they are strong enough to experience the increased force on the cells of the injured or weak areas.

The strength bounce, or actual rebound jumping, can be incorporated in an aerobic workout or strength training, or combined with the health bounce, using a two minute health bounce as a warm up and cool down.

3. **Aerobic Bounces:** This group of bounces includes jogging, sprinting, twists, jumping jacks, and other fun, creative moves. Aerobic bounces are preceeded and followed by brief health bounces to warm-up and cool-down.

Find your own pace when doing aerobic bounces and remember that rebounding places a compact force of gravity on each cell. Take your time and health bounce for a week or more prior to starting aerobic workouts to allow your internal organs to get used to the increased force of gravity on them. Make sure injured and weak areas have an opportunity to heal with the health bounce prior to aerobics.

4. **Buddy Bounces:** These assisted bounces help those who can't stand on the rebounder and bounce themselves. Sit in a chair and put your feet up on the rebounder mat and have a buddy straddle your feet and bounce. Next, sit on the rebounder and have a buddy stand behind you with feet straddling you and do the health bounce. More creative ways to

buddy bounce are described and illustrated in my *Rebounding To Better Health* book.

5. **Sitting Bounces**: These include leg lifts, bouncing "cheek-to-cheek," the V-bounce, and other creative bounces to tone the abdominals, legs, and upper body, and are actually done sitting on the rebounder mat.

It is best to rebound several times a day for short two minute sessions every day. When you are able and ready to do aerobics, one of the two minute sessions can be lengthened to a 10, 20, or 30 minute session of aerobic moves. The other two-minute sessions are best kept in the schedule, since rebounding several times each day will keep circulation, lymphatic flow, metabolism, and other body processes optimal throughout the day.

Rebounding works, and it only takes two minutes!

Suggested Rebound Program For Immune System Support

When is the best time to rebound? How many times a day is best? Rebound exercise is an everyday exercise, and the best time to rebound is all day long! Here is how easy it can be to bounce throughout the day, every day.

First thing in the morning: Health bounce for 2 minutes. Your body was under repair and did some cleansing while you slept, so this is a good time to dump the waste products that were gathered during the night, into the lymph system and flush it out of the body.

Health bounce briefly again **before going to work.** For

those who are at home or able to rebound during the day at work, health bounce for **two minutes as many times a day as possible.**

For those who leave the house to go to work, health bounce for two minutes **as soon as you get home** from work.

Health bounce **before dinner** for two minutes.

Health bounce for two minutes **during the evening several times. Health bounces every hour are ideal.**

Health bounce **before bed** for two minutes. This will not keep you awake. It will slow the brain waves to the alpha, or pre-sleep, state and enhance the chemical activity involved in the sleep mechanism.

This basic rebound program is helpful for maintaining and rebuilding health. It can be varied according to your schedule, however, consistent two minute health bounce sessions done each day keeps the lymph flowing freely, clearly, and keeps the cells healthy.

Rebounding all day every day is possible.

Aerobic Workouts

Health bouncing and aerobic workouts can be combined very effectively by gradually stretching one of your two minute health bounce sessions to a comfortable time period of 10-30 minutes and adding aerobic moves to it.

Find a time of day when you can consistently rebound daily. Start off with a two minute health bounce to warm up and then add your aerobic moves, starting with short easy segments, and increasing weekly.

Progress according to your ability, so as not to overdo. You can lengthen your session as your body gets stronger.

Adjusting your workout weekly rather than daily or every few days gives your body time to adjust to the increased activity.

End each aerobic session with the health bounce for two minutes, which flushes out toxins and the lactic acid that were created during the aerobic workout.

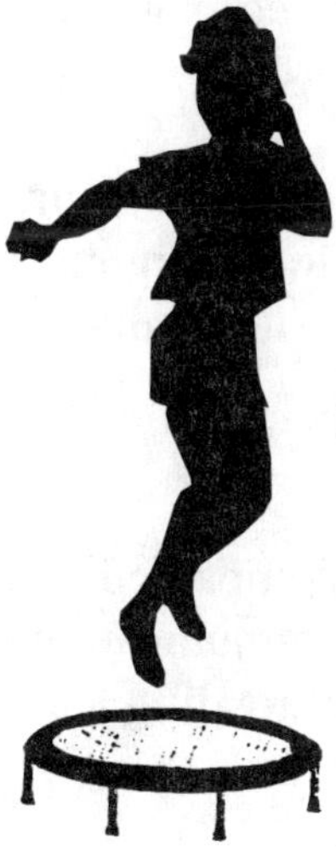

You can also get a cardiovascular workout while you do the two minute health bounce. Just put your arms in motion above the heart area as you bounce. Push hands up toward the ceiling and pull down. Then push hands out to sides, then to the front. You may add hand weights if you like. Make large circles with your arms outstretched, then small circles. Be creative and have fun.

The lymphatic system gets flushed as you bounce, or jump, or jog, or sprint, or play. Just go at your own pace and enjoy yourself!

Therapeutic Rebounding

For those who need to promote healing in the body, it is important to health bounce with feet on the mat every hour for two minutes in order to keep the lymphatic system flushed out and the white blood cell count at an optimal level.

Rebounding every hour to flush out toxins stimulates the production of more white blood cells to promote cleansing and healing. Since so many white blood cells are being used in the cleansing process, there is a natural demand for more. The white blood cell count stays high for about an hour after rebounding, then goes back to normal. This is why it is important to bounce every hour on the hour for optimal healing.

Rebounding every hour is the recommended rebounding schedule for healing injuries, colds, and flu, as well as major illnesses such as cancer, M.S., lupus, arthritis, fibromyalgia, and other concerns.

The body's innate intelligence for healing naturally is turned on by the cellular enhancement of rebounding, whether bouncing gently, or doing aerobics.

With the rebounder acting as your lymph pump, your body's number one line of defense is activated to an optimal level. Combined with the strengthening of every cell equally at the same time, amazing things happen naturally with regular rebound exercise.

When this type of rebound program is accompanied by a natural, cleansing, alkaline diet and positive communication to all the cells, **the needs of the cells are met and healing can take place in body, mind, and spirit**.

Support your body and it will protect and support you in vitality and optimal health for a long, long, time.

Rebounding For Maintenance

It is of utmost importance to aid the flow of lymph through the body every day. Since rebound exercise is the most efficient way to do that, it makes sense to rebound all day every day. That sounds impossible, however, it can be done in small amounts of time. Remember, it only takes two minutes to flush the entire lymphatic system.

Starting in the morning, it is best to health bounce as soon as you get up. Upon arising, empty the bladder and step on your rebounder for your morning wake up call. As you bounce, your body gets rid of debris from its repairs and housecleaning it did during the night. You also receive a strengthening of all your cells, plus you deliver more oxygen and blood to all your cells. Since every process of every cell is enhanced, this is a magnificent way to start your day, every day!

These two-minute bounces should be experienced as many times a day as possible, even if an aerobic workout is also done, to keep the body functioning optimally.

Rebounders belong in the workplace. Take yours to work with you. Sitting at a desk or computer for long periods of time can cause lymph to pool in the ankles and feet, bringing stiffness to these areas. Periodic two minute health bounces on the rebounder quickly moves the lymph and keeps the blood proteins from getting trapped, causing edema.

Short sessions of health bouncing keeps the immune system functioning optimally so colds, flu, and even major illnesses are avoided. Health bouncing throughout your work day also boosts metabolism, allows the burning of calories more efficiently, strengthens all cells, and enhances all body processes, which creates a balance among the systems.

Short sessions of health bouncing can be done after work, and during the evening, right up to bedtime. Don't be afraid that it will keep you awake. Rebounding slows the brainwaves, readying the body for sleep.

Rebounding every day, throughout the entire day is the ideal way to maintain your good health. The amazing thing is, that while you are maintaining good health, this cellular exercise can not do less than help you grow to an even higher level of good health.

Rebounding for your body's number one line of defense provides optimal health in all areas of your body.

Chapter Four

A Lymphatic Workout

Exercise of all kinds is known for its cardiovascular benefits, whole body strengthening and toning. I am here to tell you, though, that the immune system benefits are just as great or greater than the cardiovascular benefits, however these benefits have not been touted by aerobics instructors, trainers, or medical doctors much until now.

The focus on training and working out is beginning to change. Some personal trainers, especially those who are Certified Reboundologists, are learning to look at the entire body, mind, and spirit as one.

The human body was made to move! Movement moves lymph and lymphatic movement keeps the body healthy. Blood proteins are returned to circulation, white blood cell count is increased, and toxins leave the cells when you rebound.

Of all the different kinds of exercises, rebound exercise is the best for the lymphatic system because of the **forceful flow of lymph through the lymph veins and nodes**, and because it pulls toxins from all the cells at the same time. The entire body gets cleaner and stronger, all at once, cell by cell.

Other forms of exercise can be enhanced when combined with rebounding. A few minutes of health bouncing, jumping, or jogging combined with another form of exercise will ensure that you get the most effective lymphatic workout. **All the lymph nodes get cleansed with the more forceful flow of lymph that other forms of exercise don't supply.**

We were born to move and born to bounce. Rebound exercise is the ideal exercise. If you want to experience other forms of exercise, be sure to combine them with rebounding for optimal lymph flow and cleansing!

A two-minute health bounce before and after another form of exercise, whether it be walking, weight lifting, or others, increases circulation and oxygen to the cells, relaxes muscles, and gives that forceful flushing of the lymphatic fluid.

Exercise moves lymph. Rebound exercise moves it all at once, forcefully and efficiently!

We were born to move, and most importantly, we were born to bounce. It is cleansing, strengthening, and renewing. It enhances our natural defense systems.

Rebounding acts like a fountain of youth. It helps your body get well, and keeps it well, bounce after bounce.

Chapter Five

Natural Chelation System

In medical chelation therapy, a chelating element that has been infused into the bloodstream binds, or chelates, to heavy metals and toxins and carries them to the kidneys to be excreted. This procedure is expensive, and very invasive to the body.

The human body has its own natural chelation system. That system is the lymphatic system, since it works to pull toxins from the cells and remove them from the body.

Rebound exercise is the greatest tool to enhance the body's natural chelation process and surpasses the effectiveness of other chelation methods. This is because it works on the entire body at the same time and flushes the system with a forceful flow of lymph.

Heavy metals, stored residues from medication, toxins from the environment, and cell wastes are squeezed out of all the cells at once at the bottom of the bounce on the rebounder.

This waste material then enters the lymphatic veins that run throughout the body. At the top of the bounce on the rebounder, the change in pressure causes the one-way valves in the lymph veins to open and the lymph fluid is carried toward the heart. With continual bouncing for two minutes, the waste-filled lymph reaches circulation and is carried to the kidneys to be expelled from the body.

This is natural chelation, without any invasive material or great expense.

The key difference between natural chelation by way of rebounding to support and enhance the immune system and invasive chelation techniques is that with rebounding you get a forceful flow of lymph to effectively flush the nodes and remove toxins, and an increase in all classes of defender cells, all at once.

Some chelation methods improve cellular cleansing, but lack a way of effectively flushing out the waste. Rebound exercise, done with the simple health bounce, does both cellular cleansing and effective flushing out of the waste.

Using the rebounder for internal cleansing simplifies the cleansing process, makes it economical, and most effective, by turning on your natural chelation process inside your miraculous body.

As your rebound experience is on-going daily, so is your natural chelation process on-going, keeping your cells clean and healthy, and making a healthier you.

Chapter Six

Lymphatic Overload

While you are rebounding for better health, it is also helpful to consider whether dietary and other improvements are necessary to prevent a breakdown in immune function, caused by an overloaded lymphatic system.

Drinking purified water is important so the white blood cells aren't depleted by removing chlorine, metals and other toxins from the body. Eating pure food that is free of preservatives and chemicals also keeps the lymphatic system from being overloaded. **An overworked lymphatic system cannot efficiently remove toxins and mutated cells, which allows breakdowns in your health to take place.**

Eating fresh high fiber foods provides a natural broom to the intestinal tract to keep the hair-like villi on its lining clean and healthy. The lacteals inside these villi are the pathways of fat absorption. In a congested colon the villi can get covered over with waste and the lymphatic lacteals can't do their job effectively.

Rebound exercise helps establish a natural rhythm of gravitational pull to alleviate constipation and establish regular elimination. The villi can be restored to health and the lymphatic lacteals can function properly.

The white blood cells are responsible for removing any mutated cells that occur now and then. To make sure they are able to do that, there needs to be enough of them at the right time and place. Stressing the immune system with impure foods and water can jeopardize your health. Mutated cells that aren't removed can mutate again and become cancerous.

Eating just 6 teaspoons of sugar a day reduces the white blood cell ability by 25%. Consuming 24 teaspoons a day (below the average consumption) destroys 92% of the body's ability to destroy bacteria. This overloads your lymphatic system and compromises your entire immune system.

Protect your immune system and prevent the overloading of your lymphatic system so it can operate as it should with rebound exercise done every day, throughout the day.

Attack of the Immune System

Sometimes the immune system seems to go awry, as in an autoimmune response, and attacks certain areas of the body. In this process, antibodies actually develop against the body's own tissues.

An example of the autoimmune process is the breakdown and loss of myelin by the body's own T cells in Multiple Sclerosis. It appears that the natural defense system of the human body has actually turned against itself.

Recent research, however, shows that in M.S. a breach in the blood-brain barrier allows the T cells to enter the central nervous system and perform their damaging effects.

Any autoimmune condition is proof that the body has an imbalance or breakdown, the cause of which, is not readily apparent.

Whatever the reason for the attack of the immune system, rebound exercise can add hope, since **it affects every process of every cell with strengthening and cleaning, all the way down to the DNA, or blueprint of the body.** Regular health bouncing every day, several times a day is an ideal protocol for stimulating healing and balance within your body.

Chapter Seven

Stress, Lymphatics, and Rebounding

Studies show that stress is related to the body's ability to fight off disease. Researchers at Washington University in the U.S. reveal that exposure to chronic stress has a specific effect on immunity. Stress is related to the number of white blood cells available for defense. These studies show that persons who have experienced stress have a relatively large decrease in lymphocyte proliferation and natural killer cell activity. The longer the stress, the greater the decrease in the number of specific types of white blood cells.

White blood cells receive input from nerve fibers through which the brain regulates organs and blood vessels. Many of them produce hormones, or other signaling molecules that interact with the key stress-response areas in the brain. For example, the thymus makes hormones that are believed to influence reactions at the heart of the body's stress response.

Stress increases levels of adrenal gland hormones which, among other things, inhibits white blood cell formation and efficient functioning, and causes the thymus to shrink. Stressful conditions also lead to stimulation of the sympathetic nervous system, responsible for the fight-or-flight response. This built-in response, originally used for survival, is currently over-used because of a hectic, stressful lifestyle.

The effects of the increase of these hormones leaves the body receptive to everything from the common cold to cancer and other major illnesses.

Psychoneuroimmunology describes the interactions between emotions, the nervous system, and the immune system and offers a growing body of knowledge about the mind's effect on wellness and disease.

Everyone experiences a certain amount of stress every day. Learning to avoid some of it, and to adjust your response to it will both be helpful and healthful.

Rebounding to de-stress is a great way to protect your immune function. Rebounding relaxes the muscles and slows the brain waves to the alpha level, a pre-sleep, relaxed state. Concentrating on the fun of bouncing allows the body to relax even more.

Rebounding also strengthens all cells of all organs and brings balance to the different systems of the body.

The workplace can be very stressful. Rebounders in offices, break rooms, or on the sidelines, provide outlets for stress as employees health bounce for just two minutes at a time.

Rebounding 5-6 times a day every day reduces significantly the effects of everyday stresses. Bouncing before work and several times more after work can keep the body relaxed and the mind clear, while supporting healthy functioning and balancing of the nerves and hormones. Bouncing at the workplace is ideal.

When a stressful situation arises, stay calm and focused, and get to your rebounder as soon as you can.

Bounce and breath.

Chapter Eight

Nutritional Immune Support

Dietary habits have a great impact on immune function, for "you are what you eat," as the saying goes. Nutrient deficiency, according to the *Encyclopedia of Natural Medicine* (Prima Publishing, Ca.), is the most frequent cause of a depressed immune system.

Research is now focusing on nutrient deficiencies and the effects of too many calories, sugar, and fat. For example, the negative effects on the immune system of eating 100 grams of glucose, fructose, sucrose, honey, or orange juice start within 30 minutes, last for 5 hours, and typically include a reduction in the ability of white blood cells to destroy and engulf foreign particles at the peak of inhibition (about 2 hours after ingestion).

Research shows that after eating a cooked food meal, there is a rush of white blood cells towards the digestive system, as if the body were reacting to something harmful. Eating a raw food meal did not cause this reaction.

Overweight people seem to suffer from more infections than do those of normal weight, since experimental studies have shown that the white blood cells of overweight people were less able to destroy bacteria.

Elevated levels of cholesterol, free fatty acids, triglycerides, and bile acids inhibit the ability of white blood cells to divide, move into areas of infection, and destroy microorganisms. Alcohol has a similar effect on white blood cells, with an increased amount of alcohol consumed correlating to a greater impairment of the white blood cell mobility and function.

The modern day American diet of, high sugar, high fat, high calorie, processed fast food is not providing support for the cells of our bodies, let alone our immune systems.

Consuming basic nutritious foods as close to their nat - ural state as possible, while avoiding animal foods, white flour and sugar, hydrogenated oils, and other processed foods provides nutrition to the cells and support for the immune system.

The Three Basic Dietary Needs of the Human Body

Carbohydrates: Choose complex carbohydrates such as whole grains, brown rice, and fresh fruits and veggies, rather than simple carbohydrates such as white sugar, white pasta, white flour, and processed foods. Complex carbohydrates will provide sustained blood sugar, rather than the quick peaks and valleys you get from the simple carbos. Cancer cells feed on sugar which also adds acidity to the bloodstream and slows or inhibits the healing process. Avoid enriched and refined lifeless products.

Protein: Increase non-meat sources of protein by consuming more whole grains, seeds, nuts, beans, veggies, and soy products. **Our intestinal tract is built for fiber. Meat contains no fiber and takes hours and a lot of your energy to be digested.** Adequate protein can be received from the sources I have just mentioned. As a matter of fact, many people receive too much protein in their diets, which has a detrimental effect on the body. One negative aspect of eating too much protein is the fact that it can make the blood stream acidic. This acidity is then neutralized by calcium from the bones and teeth, which can lead to osteoporosis. Again, acidity in the bloodstream can slow or halt the healing process. The ideal pH of the bloodstream is slightly alkaline.

Fat: The cell walls of all your cells are made of 85% protein and 15% fat, so you see, you do need some nourishing fats in your body. Fat has become a scary word in relation to food, and an item some people avoid totally. **To avoid unheal-*thy* fats is advisable. To avoid *all* fat, however, can lead to health problems**. Fat is a food necessary for your health. The challenge is to figure out which fats are healthy and how much of them you need.

Unrefined, nonhydrogenated oils provide nourishing fatty acids. Avoid all hydrogenated oils, margarines, partially hydrogenated fats, and refined oils.

Fat is used as a transporter of fat soluble vitamins, good and bad cholesterol, and other fats. Fat helps the glands produce hormones, feeds the nervous system, stimulates oxidation, **enhances brain function, the immune response, and much more!** Get educated about fatty acids and stop running from fat. You need a healthy fat to even help you lose weight.

Reduce your fat intake to 20% or less of your calories from fat, then choose unrefined, or what are known as, cold-pressed oils. They have not had high heat and chemicals applied to them, nor are they stripped of nutrients. To get a supply of the different fatty acids, most people need to add omega-3 fatty acids, which are in rich supply in fresh flax seed oil. Adding a tablespoon a day to cold food, such as salad, is an excellent way to avoid a fat deficiency and feed your body to heal itself.

Your body appreciates having about two tablespoons of healthy fats each day. Flax seed oil, nuts, seeds, beans, and unrefined oils help build healthy cell walls, support for your immune system, and add vitality to your life.

Omega-three deficiencies from a lack of fresh flax seed oil in the diet contribute to, and may be the ultimate cause, nutritionally, of major diseases, including cancer. Dr. Johanna Budwig has documented over 1,000 cases of successful cancer treatment using fresh flax oil, along with other nutritional support, for over 30 years. The Gerson Clinic in Mexico also uses fresh flax seed oil, recommending two tablespoons a day for four weeks, then one tablespoon a day, thereafter.

More recent research shows that omega-3's kill human cancer cells in tissue culture without harming the normal cells present. (Breast, lung, and prostate cancer cell lines were studied.) Additional studies show that omega-3's inhibit tumor formation, including fewer tumors, smaller tumors, less metastasis (because of stronger cell walls), and longer survival time.

In terms of quantity more essential fatty acids are needed by each cell than any other nutrient. It is imperative, especially in the case of cancer, to **lower fat quantity and elevate fat quality.**

Flax seed oil should always be purchased fresh and refrigerated. One to two tablespoons a day are recommended by leading researchers and should never be heated. Consume it cold on salads, in smoothies, or take it straight.

Eating The Basics Is Eating The Best

Putting the right foods together to support your immune system can seem like a monumental task. When the focus, however, is on simplicity, cleansing and alkalinity, the process becomes easier.

When you focus on eating foods as close to their natural state as possible, you eliminate chemicals and artificial additives that could place a burden on your immune system. Focus on purity and whole foods as you learn to eliminate foods that read as chemical sets or contain high and unhealthy fat content, and are high in sugar.

Next, remove the table sugar, which is just empty cal--ories, and replace it with Splenda, which comes from sugar, but has been safely transformed and doesn't affect the blood sugar level.

By removing animal products, junk food, and sugar products, your diet will provide less acidity to the bloodstream, making it easier for your healing to take place. The ideal diet contains 80% of foods that leave an alkaline-ash and 20% of foods leaving an acid-ash after digestion. Consuming alkalizing fresh vegetables, fruits, whole grains, nuts and seeds, predominately, will provide this ratio of alkaline/ash foods.

Juicing fresh vegetables and fruits gives you condensed nutrients that will drive toxins from the cells and provide superior nourishment for healing. These juices need no digestion, and take less energy for assimilation than solid foods. Foods eaten raw provide synergistic nutritionals with enzymes intact.

Consuming an abundance of fresh raw salads or juices provides opportunities to add flax seed oil to the diet. A tablespoon or two as part of the dressing, or added into the juice are easy ways to consume it without taking it straight.

Make sure grains truly are whole grains and not enriched, or refined. Add them to salads with raw almonds or other nuts and soy cheese for added nutrition and variety.

Select organic foods when possible for higher quality, more nutritious foods. Focus on simplicity, purity, and creativity and get accustomed to the superior diet that will help feed you into wellness. Just remember to look forward to foods you *can* have, instead of those you *can't* have.

Real Foods Shopping List

The following list was designed to help people choose healthy foods that also have a good flavor. It is not all inclusive, so explore all you want. This list is a guideline to help you make a transition into healthier eating without venturing into disappointing flavors.

Cereals: Avoid enriched, refined grains, sugar, hydrogenated oils. Choose cereals from a variety of grains. Arrowhead Mills, Barbara's, Nature's Path, Health Valley are excellent choices.

Pasta: Avoid refined, enriched grains. Choose Quinoa, spelt, amaranth (all contain more protein than wheat), brown rice, corn. Health Valley, Ancient Harvest, Vita Spelt, Arrowhead Mills. Also in bulk in some stores.

Rice: Avoid white rice. Basmati brown rice, Lundberg special aromatic rices are a treat!

Nut Butters: Avoid sugar and hydrogenated oils. Choose organic freshly ground, Arrowhead Mills, Deaf Smith, Nu-Value.

Milk: No dairy. Choose soy or rice milk. Silk has best taste, also Rice Dream, Edensoy, Westsoy,

Sweeteners: Avoid white and brown sugar. Choose Splenda, concentrated frozen fruit juice, fruit puree, brown rice syrup, raw honey, barley malt syrup, maple syrup, unsulphured molasses.

Beverages: Choose filtered water, herbal teas, 100% fruit and vegetable juices. Knudsen, After-The-Fall, and Santa Cruz juices, and Celestial Seasonings teas taste good. Avoid caffeine, "juice- ades," "blends," or "drinks," and carbonation.

Fats and Oils: Avoid hydrogenated and partially hydrogenated fats. Choose unrefined oils like extra-virgin olive oil, **flax seed oil**, butter. Spectrum, Arrowhead Mills, Barleans are good brands.

Bread: Avoid sugar, enriched white flour, hydrogenated oils, and chemicals. Choose Ezekiel, Alvarado Street, Food For Life sprouted grain breads, buns, and tortillas.

Cookies and Snacks: No sugar, white flour, or hydrogenated oils. Choose whole grains, fruit-juice sweetener, aluminum-free baking powder. Barbara's, Nature's Warehouse, Pamela's, Health Valley are good examples.

Packaged Mixes: Avoid hydrogenated oil, sugar, white flour, MSG, preservatives, artificial flavors and colors. Choose Fantastic Foods Burger Mixes and other products, Barbara's, Seeds Of Change rice mixes and sauces.

Frozen foods: Avoid white pasta, hydrogenated oils, preservatives, and MSG. Choose Boca Organic Burgers, Natural Touch Organic Burgers and Okara Patties, Amy's dinners, burgers, and pizzas, Rice Dream Ice Cream.

Cheese Substitutes: Lisinatti Almond cheese (great!), Lite & Less Parmesan (soy), Galaxy Cheese Veggie Cheese slices and shreds in many flavors (excellent).

Seasonings: Bragg's Liquid Amino Acids, Dr. Bronner's Mineral Broth, Vegit. Top salads with Bragg's, flax oil and herbs.

Salad Dressings: Avoid sugar, hydrogenated oils, and preservatives. Choose Annies Naturals, Simply Delicious, Cook's Classic, Nasoya, Newman's Own.

Water: Filtered by reverse osmosis or distillation, **never from the tap.** Drink 2/3 ounce for each pound of body weight daily.

Nutrients For Immune Support

Vitamin A: Stimulates or enhances immune processes such as induction of anti-tumor activity, white blood cell function, and increase of antibody response. Vitamin A has also significant antiviral activity and has prevented the immune suppression induced by adrenal hormones, and stress-induced shrinkage of the thymus gland. Vitamin A stores typically plummet during the course of an infection.

Vitamin A rich foods include green vegetables, the most plentiful being carrots and hot chili peppers, barley grass juice and alfalfa sprouts. Chlorella, a single-cell edible algae, besides being high in vitamin A, also contains nutrients known as "youth factors."

Carotenes: The most widespread group of naturally occurring pigments in nature, 30-50 varieties having vitamin A activity. Research shows that carotenes exert many immune system enhancing effects independent of vitamin A activity.

High carotene content can be found in green leafy vegetables, and orange-yellow fruits and vegetables. Legumes, grains and seeds are also significant sources.

Flavonoids: Another group of plant pigments that act as antioxidants that protect against free-radical damage.

Citrus fruits, legumes, berries, green tea, and parsley are good sources.

Vitamin C: Antibacterial, antiviral and antioxidant, with effects such as enhanced white blood cell response and function, increased interferon levels, increased secretion of thymic hormones, and improved integrity of mucous membrane linings.

Citrus fruits, tomatoes, green peppers, broccoli, parsley, dark green leafy vegetables, peas, cantaloupe, strawberries, cabbage, potatoes, and asparagus are excellent sources.

Vitamin E: An antioxidant with free-radical protection, and helps protect against tumor growth.

Vitamin E is available in cold-processed plant oils, egg yolk, nuts and seeds, whole grains, and green leafy vegetables.

Zinc: Promotes the destruction of foreign particles and microorganisms, acts as a protectant against free-radical damage, acts synergistically with vitamin A, is required for proper white blood cell function, and is necessary in activating serum thymic factor — a hormone with immune enhancing properties.

Good sources include whole grains, legumes, and eggs.

Selenium: Enhances the expression of Interleukin-II, the rate of white blood cell proliferation and differentiation into forms capable of killing tumor cells and microorganisms.

Onions are high in selenium, with potatoes, tomatoes, carrots, and cabbage also having good selenium value.

Botanicals: Echinacea and astragalus have antiviral, antibacterial, properties with profound immune enhancing effects.

Taheebo tea: antibacterial, antiviral, and antifungal properties from the Purple Lapacho tree.

Colloidal silver: Antibacterial, antiviral, antifungal properties safely suffocate microorganisms and support your immune system.

Pure water: Chlorine and fluoride and other impurity residues can overload the immune system. Drink only purified water. Reverse osmosis and distilled are good sources. Never tap water.

This list of nutrients for immune support is far from complete, for all vitamins and minerals work synergistically in the body. Since a natural balance of nutrients is necessary, all attempts to get your nutrition from foods in their natural state should be made, with a natural harmony of vitamins and minerals as they are manufactured in the whole food, rather than as some human's formula for vitamin/mineral supplementation.

Eating a wide variety of fresh fruits and vegetables, nuts, seeds, and whole grains, with soy foods as good sources of protein, provides a balance of nutrients and keeps the body slightly on the alkaline edge where healing and good health can manifest.

Rebounding and Nutrition

Rebound exercise, being a cellular exercise, enhances all processes of the body. Taking in pure, fresh nutrients from foods as close to their natural state as possible feeds the cells of the body, and synergistically, rebounding helps the cells utilize these nutrients.

Digestion is enhanced, organs of the endocrine system are improved, becoming more productive, assimilation of nutrients becomes more efficient, and transit time through the intestinal tract is shortened as elimination improves.

Less toxins are stored throughout the body as digestion and elimination improve, allowing the immune system to perform more efficiently, as it becomes less and less overloaded.

Metabolism is boosted with rebound exercise, enhancing fat burning and energy production. Rebounding for short periods of time, such as two minutes each, five to six times a day supports the immune system in many ways, one of them being in improved processing of food and delivery of nutrients to the cells, and keeping the cells and lymph fluid clear of extra toxic waste.

A couple of minutes of health bouncing before and after each healthy meal is ideal activity for improved immune support. Feed your cells optimally, and rebound, rebound, rebound to turn on their ability to heal themselves and stay well.

Beyond The Physical

For as he thinketh in his heart, so is he…

Proverbs 23:7

Chapter Nine

Emotions and Immunity

You are more than what you eat. You are the result, additionally, of every thing you think and feel. Research is now showing that what goes on in the brain can interact with the immune system to suppress it or enhance it. Nerve cells connect the thymus directly to the hypothalamus and white blood cells respond directly to some of the same chemicals that carry messages from cell to cell.

Scientists who have traced a pathway from the brain to the immune cells have proved that "negative emotions can stop white blood cells dead in their tracks." (www.hps-online.com)

The central nervous system has branches with nerve endings that terminate in the glands which regulate the immune system, providing constant biofeedback between hormones and neurochemicals, or peptides, which are messenger molecules that carry information from perception to the brain, to cells, and back again. Your immune system, therefore, functions like a sensory organ that responds to external stimuli from the nervous system.

"Peptide transmitters produced by the immune system function as a sort of sixth sense, supplementing the information the brain receives from the other five senses and possibly accounting for the way some people sense that something is wrong before they actually get sick," according to Dr. Bernie Siegel, *in Peace, Love & Healing.*

Approximately sixty known peptide molecules, some of which have familiar names, like endorphins, interleukens, and interferon turn feelings into chemicals and link the mind to the physical.

As mentioned in Chapter 7, the action triggered by our fight-or-flight mechanism in early days of man used up the extra adrenaline and other adrenal related chemicals, and calmness returned to the body shortly after the fight-or-flight incident occurred.

The same biochemical responses to fight-or-flight are triggered today hundreds of times throughout the day, however, the stimulative hormones, extra glucose, and other aneurochemicals released into the blood are not utilized by fast, physical action. Negative emotions are repressed, and the fight-or-flight stimulatives wreak havoc on the immune system, even withering away lymph nodes. Within one day, any uncontrolled stress lowers the efficiency of the immune system's killer cells.

Calming, soothing, neurochemicals, similarly, stimulate secretion of calming, soothing hormones. Dr. Michael Weiner, in *Maximum Immunity*, says, "By learning how to control our mind, subtle hormonal changes emerge that can then control our biochemical reality."

Dr. Bernie Siegel, Yale University's cancer surgeon, adds, "psychological and spiritual development are capable of reversing the disease process."

According to Louise Hay, author of *You Can Heal Your Body*, the mental thought patterns of criticism, anger, resentment, and guilt cause the most "dis"-ease in our bodies. Physical symptoms are only an outer effect of our thoughts.

Common expressions such as "He's a pain in the neck, Get off my back, I'm kicking myself, and It's eating me up inside," directly affect the body's tissues. In essence, your cells understand your verbal language, and respond to it with negative, or positive physical effects.

Positive thought patterns and expressions, lead to positive changes of health and vitality through an enhanced immune system.

Researcher Candace Pert says, "I can no longer make a distinction between the brain and the body....Indeed, the more we know about neuropeptides, the harder it is to think in the traditional terms of a mind and body. It makes more sense to speak of a single, integrated entity, a bodymind."

"The brain is not just for thinking; it is a survival organ." (Albert Szent-Györgyi)

Rebounding, Emotions, and Immunity

Regular exercise has been shown to enhance mood-elevating chemicals in the brain called endorphins. People who exercise tend to have a more positive outlook and an enhanced self-esteem. One of the greatest benefits of exercise is the release of tension, anxiety, and pent-up feelings.

Rebound exercise supplies these benefits and more to the body, in an enhanced, fun way, without the strain of some of the regular exercises.

Rebounding is relaxing, which triggers the parasympathetic system to produce chemicals that are calming, soothing, and relaxing. In slowing the brain waves to the alpha state, the body remains calm, meditative, and the immune system is supported.

Rebounding grounds you to the earth's energy, allowing your natural chi energy to flow freely, which supports optimal immune functions. A grounded, relaxed body gives the body an alkaline edge toward healing by balancing systems and enhancing the activity of every cell at once.

Rebounding for emotional health is easy and effective by doing the health bounce for 1-2 minutes several times a day. This enhances the production of brain chemicals that elevate mood, stimulates neuropeptide delivery of positive emotions to the cells in the biofeedback loop, and provides an opportunity for positive communication with your body.

Rebounding is fun, so thinking thoughts that contribute to health and healing can be an easy task. When making a conscious effort to change your thought patterns and feelings, rebounding is extremely helpful. "Dumping," or letting go of out-moded thoughts and feelings is enhanced because of the cellular cleansing, strengthening of brain cells, and enhancement of neuropeptides and brain chemicals stimulated by the increased pull of gravity on every cell at the same time. Consequently, new thought patterns can be established by repeating them while bouncing.

The immune system is supported by the flushing of lymph, cleansing of lymph nodes, and increase of white blood cells, however, the grounding, relaxing, and positive biofeedback are just as important benefits to healthy immunity.

Emotions don't happen to you, you choose them, and the point of power is in the present moment. Making a conscious choice to pay more attention to your thoughts and emotions, and how you express them is a beginning to giving your body's defense system more support.

Think On Me

Think on me.
Know me well.
I can heal you
And bring you great joy.
Be one,
Be well,
As my light streams in.
Think on me often,
Become more like me —
Joyous, bold in love.
Take your day lightly.
All that matters is love.
Let it flow out and back,
In ever greater flow.
You are well.
Think on me.
Remember.

~Linda Brooks

Chapter 10

Spirituality and Immune Support

Deep within your core there is an energy of infinite intelligence. It is this awesome energy known as spirit that has baffled scientists as they have watched individuals in what they called "terminal" situations show signs of miraculous, unexplained healing.

Why is it that regular church attendees are more likely to live healthy lives? Why do people who pray and are prayed for get well faster than those who are not prayed for?

Answers to these questions are not easily answered from a scientific point of view. True health and healing starts from within, in that unlimited creative intelligence, known as Spirit, God, Divine Being, that power greater than ourselves, yet living in us, making us one with it.

Recognizing our oneness with this ultimate power ignites the energy of this infinite intelligence in every cell, every molecule of our being, and it manifests as health, sometimes beyond our wildest dreams.

No part of the human body operates as an island. When spiritual DNA information is activated, the blueprint for perfection is broadcast through the body, as light, love and truth.

I do not profess to have all the answers relative to spirituality and immune support and healing. Nor do I intend to speak of a specific "religious" viewpoint. I merely am coming from a point of awe when it comes to exploring the possibilities that the healing force of God within us can express in our spiritual human bodies.

Dr. Edward Taub, known as America's Wellness Medical Doctor, says that total health rejuvenation "requires stimulating your own natural healing force, which is equivalent to the presence of God in every one of your trillions of cells. Medical science defines the 'healing force' as 'merely an array of polypeptide chemicals such as endorphins and enkephalins,' so no wonder your healing force beguiles physicians who search in all the wrong places and ask the wrong questions.... stimulating your healing force — begins deep inside you, at the level of your soul, and radiates outward."

That healing force of truth and love triggers the positive chemicals that support the immune functions to their fullest. It is ignited by prayerful connection with the inner intelligence running deep within, and among, all your cells.

Dr. Harold Koenig, of Duke University Medical Center, says, "Preliminary evidence suggests religious patients have lower levels of cortisol, the stress chemical that damages the heart. The components of their immune systems are more plentiful. They exercise more and smoke or drink less."

He goes on to say, "Furious attempts to gain control over health situations breed anxiety and depression. But religious beliefs provide 'an indirect form of control' that helps interrupt the vicious cycle." Dr. Koenig's research on 850 hospital patients showed better results when stress management included religion.

Again, the point of power is in the present moment. The here and now moment is in alignment with God, or higher power, our healing force. Our higher power, healing force, is here, now, so our awareness of the present allows us access to the love and truth and healing power available within us.

Thinking on yesterday and tomorrow pulls us away from the truth and love in today.

Rebounding, Spirituality, and Immunity

Rebound exercise is a very spiritual experience! I believe this powerful statement is true, however, I have no scientific data to offer as "proof."

Your entire being encompasses body, mind, and spirit, and since rebounding affects every aspect of every cell, it stands to reason that it affects the physical body, emotions, and the spirit.

The process of rebounding from a spiritual level begins with relaxation of muscles, and the slowing of the brain waves to the alpha level. The shock-free bounce provides grounding so your chi energy flows freely through your energy centers and meridian points.

Your immune system is supported and enhanced by the two-minute health bounce and by the natural connection to the core of your inner being. Your perfection is being remembered by every cell, bounce after bounce.

That little kid in you wants to bounce and play as the realization of your truth runs through your systems. The spirit part of you that is also connected to all other parts of you and everything around you begins to vibrate with a feeling of enhanced well-being and joy.

Your body systems seek balance and your mind and spirit seek oneness with your physical body. Your body is a miracle fulfilled through your spirit. Your Soft-Bounce rebounder is the tool that stimulates your body's ability to heal itself.

Verbal or silent prayer, meditation, visualization, and affirmations are tools that you can use while you do your easy, relaxing bounces, connected with Spirit in the moment.

"When we can gather the courage and take one more step beyond our perceived limits, what we will discover is that there is still ground beneath our feet."

~~Al Secunda
(The Fifteen Second Principle)

Chapter 11

Stories of Success

I have received countless comments and stories from people who have received benefits of natural healing and wanted to share them with me. I will now pass along to you a few of them having to do with immune function.

I will begin with a brief story from Celeste, whose full story can be read in one of my upcoming books on rebounding and M.S. I met Celeste when I went to B.C. to teach my Certified Reboundologist workshop and she became one of my graduates. The whole group sat in awe and applauded her as she actually was able to give a jump off the mat unassisted.

She picked me up at the airport in her hot pink wheelchair, drove us home, then walked up the stairs to bed, something she could not have done six months earlier.

Celeste's Story

"I was diagnosed with M.S. in 1995 after many years of frustration with varying symptoms that were dismissed by my doctors as, "Oh you are working too hard, you have to learn to manage your stresses better," or even after I went legally blind in my left eye in 1986 and legally blind in both eyes in 1991, "you just need some time off work."

Other major symptoms were: loss of use of my bladder in 1991, extreme fatigue for many years, ringing in my ears, extreme nausea, anxiety, panic attacks, insomnia, extreme vertigo, loss of balance, tremors, bumping into walls and door frames, numbness and tingling in the extremities, disorientation, and cognitive problems.

After receiving all the bad and none of the good from prescribed medication, I decided to take a holistic approach to my health and well-being and I am sure glad I did. On this regime I have progressed from being 95% in bed or in a wheelchair to 95% out of the wheelchair!

Exercise is essential daily, many times a day in fact. The exercise I found to be the most effective to remove toxins and exercise every cell in my body is a cellular exercise called rebound exercise, which can be done even if you can't stand up. I couldn't stand properly or even sit up long enough to eat my dinner when I started rebounding in 1996. My husband lifted me out of my wheelchair and held me on the rebounder.

One of the first benefits I noticed was that my balance improved greatly. Then I got more energy, my legs came more alive and felt stronger, less numb and tingly, I was less dizzy, and generally overall felt much more energy, less stressed and alive again.

I started with about 10 seconds and worked up to two minutes after two years. On the third year I could do three minutes, and one minute of that was with my feet leaving the mat. Wow!!! I was on my way!!!

I am currently rebounding five to six times a day. At the top of the bounce you are momentarily weightless. During this brief transition of weightlessness and back to gravity the health benefits are taking place at the cellular level. Your bones and muscles react as if they are holding a weight, yet there is no strain. At the bottom of the bounce the cells experience a gentle squeezing, stimulating the lymphatic system to get working to remove toxins, increase white blood cell count, and stimulate every cell to become stronger."

~~ Celeste Veld, British Columbia
(Celeste also did internal cleansing, natural diet, and supplements.)

Many Benefits For Janise

"I definitely have fewer and less frequent respiratory problems than I had before I started rebounding in August, 1994. If I rebound regularly (3 to 4 times per week for 30 minutes per session), my sciatica pain is much less and I can do much more strenuous activity without having to worry about my back.

I've also found that on several occasions, I was able to beat an illness with rebounder activity. Sometimes I would catch something just before a show (to demonstrate and sell rebounders). By the end of the first day of the show, after demonstrating the rebounder all day, staying on it for at least five or six hours with some breaks — mainly just health bouncing — whatever was trying to make me ill simply disappeared! I've never developed a full blown illness after a show, and I was also able to keep my energy up during the whole show."

~~~Janise Baldo-Pulaski, New Mexico

Maria's MS Story

I met Maria when I went to Canada, after she called me to request a Certified Reboundologist workshop in her town of Edmonton, Alberta, since she was very happy that rebound exercise had helped her body heal itself from MS.

"When I was 18 years old, I was diagnosed with possibly having Multiple Sclerosis. By age 24, it was confirmed through a Spinal Tap (a conclusive test at that time).

I had a very bad episode with my M.S., causing me to have numbness in my limbs, dizziness, staggered speech and walking, unending fatigue, loss of coordination, headaches, and temporary loss of almost all my vision. I was never so
~~~

afraid in my life! I was put on steroids. After using them for a short time and experiencing side effects, I decided to try alternative measures.

My chiropractor suggested I use rebound exercise with a temporary cleansing diet, and supplements to help strengthen my immune system. Within months, I noticed a significant improvement in my overall health. I have used rebound exercise for several years now and feel healthier and more fit than ever.

I truly believe that rebounding has made my immune system, muscles, joints, etc., very strong and has helped me to get on with my life."

~~~Maria Herperger, Edmonton, Alberta

No Surgery For Louise!

"In December, 1991, a car hit me in the right front fender, messing up my right shoulder and tendons and ligaments in my right arm. In spite of physical therapy three times a week, the medical department at work thought that I might aggravate the condition by working, so I was put on disability and had six months to recover or take permanent disability.

My doctor wanted me to have an operation and retire. I continued physical therapy and started seeing a chiropractor and acupuncturist. I couldn't tell if any of these were helping, and my six months of disability were about to end.

My chiropractor believed in the rebounder. I faithfully began bouncing daily, and in four weeks I could bounce for 20 minutes at a time.

The doctor was surprised at my recovery and signed the papers to release me to return to work. A medical department nurse's eyes popped and her mouth opened wide with
~~~

disbelief as I came walking into medical. I fooled them all, and I owe it all to the rebounder.

It is June, 2003 and I am still working with no problems from my shoulder and right tendons and ligaments. I tell people who have pain in their joints to get them a rebounder. That is the secret."

~~~Louise Southern, Kentucky

No More Allergies, Colds, or Flu!

"Since I have been rebounding for three to four years, it is rare that I have any illness bother me. I have had no flu in that time, my allergies are gone, and if I feel like something is trying to get me, I just get on my rebounder often, and it goes away.

As an educator, I am often around people who are sick, and it doesn't affect me, since rebounding boosts my immune system."

~~~Dave VanWhervin, Michigan

Dry Eye Better

"I had a dry condition in one eye that caused it to tear up often. I started rebounding about two years ago, and my dry eye got better."

~~~Sharon Woods, Ohio

Rebounded After Surgery

"After having surgery for a torn ligament in my knee, I was back on my rebounder within a couple of days doing a
~~~

gentle health bounce. By the second week I was able to do some light running. The rebounding not only helped keep the inflammation out of my knee so it could heal, it also helped with the nauseous feeling I experienced as a result of the anesthetic and pain killers I had received during and after the surgery. It seemed to work the residuals of these medications out of my body.

I have been rebounding for three years and no longer have colds, flu, sore throat or viruses."

~~~Joyce Green, Michigan

Yearly Colds and Flu Gone!

"Since rebounding for the last 2 1/2 years, I have had no major colds or flu. I used to get them at least once a year, and sometimes twice. If I feel a little under the weather, I get rid of it quickly by rebounding."

~~~Martha Miners, Washington

MS Better at 82!

"I am 82, with MS, and after I had been rebounding for just three months, my doctor told me that I was walking much better."

~~~Mrs. Sampson, Michigan

Vertigo Gone!

"When I started using the rebounder my vertigo problems virtually left. By just doing the health bounce, I have had no major episodes and rarely have any problems at all with vertigo, because if I feel one coming on I can rebound and it leaves.
~~~

My friend came to visit from out of town, with feet so swollen she was using a walker. I got her on my Soft-Bounce rebounder and she did a 2-minute health bounce off and on several times a day. She was so amazed that the swelling in her feet and knees was going down that she would pop on the rebounder very often and bounce. In about three days the swelling was gone and she went home without using her walker."

Donna Saunders, Michigan

Healing Leads To Rebound Performance

"About three years ago I began rebounding for the nerve damage on the sides of my legs. As my body got cleaner and stronger I was able to dance and play on my rebounder, doing high kicks and other fun dance steps. I now enjoy giving rebound performances dressed in cowgirl, and other fun costumes that coordinate with the music and dance.

I am also happy that I no longer get colds and cold sores, have no more sinus problems and itching in my ears, thanks to the rebounder. My eyes also improved so I am not required to wear glasses when I drive!"

~~~Cindy Peńa, Michigan

Smoking Detoxification

"I used the rebounder almost every morning for as long as I can remember. After I quit smoking, one morning I kept on rebounding till I worked up a good sweat, and you would not believe the stench! The whole house smelled awful from the detoxing of stored toxins from smoking. I have rebounded on a regular basis ever since — about 25 years."

~~~Raymond, Ohio

Weight Loss, and More

"Before I started rebounding about 10 months ago, I was more than 35 pounds heavier. Rebounding helped me drop the weight and clean out my system. I am not sick, even when I am around sick people, and have a greater all-over feeling of well-being."

~~~Solomon Pryor, Michigan

Injury From Fall Better

"Rebounding for a minute or two at a time with hand weights helped strengthen my shoulder, upper arm, wrist and hand after a fall. Rebounding makes me feel positive when it keeps my joints clean."

~~~Shirley Cridland, Ontario

Rebounding Favorable To Immune System

In addition, I will add how rebounding helped get rid of the periodic edema in my mother's legs, ankles, and feet. I pushed the rebounder under her feet, as she sat up in a chair, and stood in the middle of the mat and health bounced for 2-4 minutes several times a day. Within days, a week at the most, the swelling was completely gone, and circulation improved.

I had so many physical and emotional toxins stored in my cells from childhood and early adult life, that it took me several years to clear them out. A few years ago, with a major change in my life, I had a brief ear infection. I jumped high on my rebounder to move the lymph fluid with force and pump it out of the inner ear and send white blood cells in to clean up infection. I also affirmed that I had no need of this condition on any level and expected it to leave and not return. It worked!

Knowledge Is Power

"Knowledge...is not always power unless Wisdom is used in the application of same."

~~~Edgar Cayce Reading 262-104

Chapter 12

Taking Action

Where do you go from here? The Vitally Yours program for cellular health is bottom line truth and hopefully, it makes sense to you. The next step is for you to apply this knowledge and make necessary changes in your lifestyle that lead you to greater health and vitality.

This knowledge, when applied, helps your body heal itself, which is a pretty powerful concept. Armed with knowledge, you can now take responsibility for your health.

On a scale of 1 to 10, where 1 represents an unhealthy lifestyle of fast-food, junk food nutrition, no exercise, couch potato lifestyle, and 10 represents optimal nutrition, daily rebound exercise, plus positive emotions and an uplifting spiritual attitude, estimate where your lifestyle falls. It is an individual process. Make no judgment about where you think you are on the 1 to 10 scale, just recognize it as your starting point and know that you will continue from there at your own speed, and according to your inner guidance.

Of all the wonderful benefits of rebound exercise, the greatest overall benefit is the way it brings homeostasis to the body on all levels of spirit, mind, and the physical body. Balance among the body's systems, many internal processes, organs, tendons, bones, and tissues, along with the connection of feelings with body and spirit, reaches a point of truth in your whole being, moving cellular health toward optimal wellness.

The information in this book about your body's ability to heal itself with such simple, natural means is not typical. It is unusually simple, and yet it works, when understood, believed, and applied to your life.

Work from the inside out and help your immune system do its job proudly, instead of being compromised by invasive techniques that can act as band-aids, confusing and upsetting the body's natural balance.

Get excited, and expect to be well by visualizing yourself well, and thinking only health. Listen to your body as you progress. Know you are well, and give your body the opportunity to respond to that knowing! Wishing and hoping leaves room for doubt in your cells. Plant only positive, sure seeds. Know you are well, and bounce that message simultaneously to all of your 75 trillion cells.

"When we learn something about the human mechanism — and particularly the mind which controls it — there are no limits to the heights we can climb." (Ben Sweetland, *I Can! The Key To Life's Golden Secrets*)

Your body is the miracle! The Soft-Bounce rebounder is the perfect tool to help it transform into health and vitality by enhancing your number one line of defense and giving you hundreds of other benefits.

Now you know more truth. Let it free you to confidently and lovingly take more responsibility for your health.

"And you will know the truth, and that very truth will make you free." (John 8:32)

Just imagine people bouncing and jumping their way into a more joyful and meaningful world through less illness and toxicity.

The rebounder is the perfect tool to bring out the miracles in your perfect body.

Chapter 13

Maintaining Balance

The main objective of rebound exercise is to bring the body into homeostasis, or the balance of systems where everything is synergistically operating in equilibrium.

Balance within your body from a program that meets the basic needs of the cells is enhanced by a lifestyle that has a balance of activities that support your healthy lifestyle.

Taking time for family fun, relaxation, and quiet time, is just as important as the time spent at work. Balance on the inside should reflect balance on the outside and vice versa.

Changing your mind changes your body. Changing your mind also means changing some habits, like shopping and exercising and learning mechanisms to cope with and alleviate stress.

Changing habits takes time and being patient with yourself. Listen to your body and feel its need to slow down, journal, take more action, or recognize needed activities.

Coming into balance requires that you learn to love and value yourself as God does. Taking control of your health and life means looking with awe at your potential to create, grow, and heal.

Little do we know what we are truly capable of achieving, and the closer we get to looking at our potential in spirit, mind, and body from a point of love and oneness with Divine Mind, the closer we get to realizing our purpose: to return to the heart of God by loving each other and feeling loved, unconditionally.

"Health, real health, is from within and does not have to be manufactured in the without. It is the normal condition of man, a condition true to the reality of his being."

~~~Charles Fillmore

~~~References And Product Information

~~~Notes~~~

It only takes two minutes of health bouncing to flush the lymphatic tubes and triple the white blood cell count."

References

Brooks, Linda, Cancer — *A Simple Approach,* Ohio: Vitally Yours Press, 2002.

Brooks, Linda, *Rebounding To Better Health*, Nebraska: KE Publishing, Fourth Printing 2001.

Brooks, Linda, *Rebounding and Your Lymphatic System*, Ohio: Vitally Yours Press, 2000.

Carter, Albert E., *The New Miracles of Rebound Exercise,* Arizona: Nature Distributors, 1988.

Garrison, Robert H., JR., Elizabeth Somer, *The Nutrition Desk Reference,* Connecticut: Keats Publishing, 1985.

Guyton, Arthur C., M.D., *Textbook of Medical Physiolo*gy, 7th edition, Philadelphia: W. B. Saunders Co., 1986.

Hay, Louise L., *Heal Your Body*, California: Hay House, Inc., 1984.

Lamb, Kevin, *"Faith, not laughter, may be the best medicine,"* Ohio: Dayton Daily News: April 25, 2003.

Murray, Michael, N.D., Pizzorno, Joseph, N.D., *Encyclopedia of Natural Medicine*, California: Prima Publishing, 1998.

Siegel, Bernie S., M.D., *Love, Medicine and Miracles,* New York: Harper and Row, 1986.

Siegel, Bernie S., M.D., *Peace, Love and Healing*, New York: Harper and Row, 1989.

Schwartz, Jack, *It's Not What You Eat, But What Eats You*, California: Celestial Arts, 1988.

Sweetland, Ben, *"I Can" The Key to Life's Golden Secrets*, New York: Cadillac Publishing Co., Inc., 1953.

Taub, Edward A., M.D., *Balance Your Body, Balance Your Life*, New York: Kensington Publishing Corp., 1999.

Trowbridge, Bob, M. Div., *The Hidden Meaning of Illness*, Virginia: A.R.E. Press, 1996.

Weiner, Michael, M.D., *Maximum Immunity*, www.hps-online.com.

www.berkeleywellness.com.

www.eucerin.co.uk/skin/physio-7.html.

NEEDAK® Soft-Bounce™Rebounder

A true rebounder is not a toy. It is a piece of exercise equipment designed to promote your body's natural healing. Rebounding will not jeopardize your health in any way, when a quality unit like the Soft-Bounce rebounder is selected and used properly.

Needak Manufacturing, in O'Neill Nebraska has been making the highest quality units since 1990. These units have been tested well in the marketplace and carry a limited lifetime warranty.

The secret to a truly soft, safe bounce is in the durable, 4-inch long, specially coiled springs that give a shock-free bounce with less of your effort. Models with 2-inch springs provide jarring at the bottom of the bounce that can cause damage to joints and back.

Spring loaded legs fold inside the frame, and the frame folds in half, and slips into a durable carrying bag for transport in a car, or as baggage on a plane.

The portable stabilizer bar used for balance and safety fits conveniently on the legs of the rebounder and adjusts to three heights. It is great for seniors, beginners, children, and aerobics.

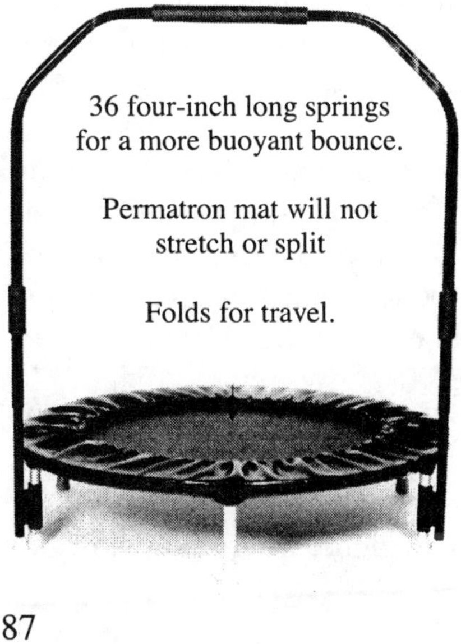
36 four-inch long springs
for a more buoyant bounce.
Permatron mat will not
stretch or split
Folds for travel.

Book, video, and instructions included.

Product specials and free shipping: 877-299-9547, or 937-456-9633, or www.2rebound.com

Rebounding Books

Cancer — A Simple Approach, by Linda Brooks — A comprehensive program of cleansing, feeding, and exercising the cells to fully activate the immune system and utilize the body's own healing power through a simple, non-invasive approach, including specifics for spirit, mind, body healing. **$5.95**

Rebounding To Better Health, A Practical Guide to The Ultimate Exercise, by Linda Brooks — A simple, practical guide on rebounding and various health conditions as well as aerobics objectives, with photos, illustrations, and success stories from rebound lovers of all walks of life. **$5.95**

Rebounding and Your Immune System, by Linda Brooks — A basic book on your body's defense system and how rebound exercise enhances its efficiency so your body can heal itself. Illustrations, lymphatic terminology, and therapeutic rebound moves are included. **$7.95**

Rebound Videos

Bounce Before You Jump, An Introduction To Rebound Movement, by Linda Brooks — The first how-to video with safe rebound techniques, workouts for beginner, intermediate, and advanced levels that shows how and when to do moves, weight loss tips, therapy, aerobics, sports, and senior moves. **$19.95**

What Comes After The Bounce? By Linda Brooks — Take the guesswork out of your start-up rebounding, keep it fun, find your beginning threshold, learn when and how long to bounce, and build your personal rebounding program, safely and effectively. **$19.95**

A Beginner's Rebound Workout, by Linda Brooks — A safe, easy-to-follow, beginner's rebound routine designed for whole body toning, weight loss, and increased vitality. Warm up, beginner's aerobics, slow down, and cool down. **$19.95**

VITAL HEALTH NEWS

A newsletter for body, mind, and spirit with a back-to-basics approach to cellular health.

Linda's uplifting approach has inspired hundreds of individuals on their paths to greater health and fulfillment since 1988. Enjoyment of greater health is now as close as your mailbox. Subscribe today, and be inspired by:

Rebound cellular exercise - creative routines, success stories, interviews about rebounding, senior news, educational rebound articles in ***Your Amazing Body section,*** with new rebound product announcements, specials, and much more!

Food for your cells - check ***The Nutrition Corner*** for vegetarian recipes, discussions with health care practitioners, the basics on internal cleansing, shopping tips, the truth about your food and your health, new product news, and more.

Motivation and Inspiration - ***The Real Good News*** for spiritual growth, taking charge of your health, and lifestyle enhancement, including motivational messages of truth and love that have made Linda's newsletter grow in popularity year after year!

"Your newsletter is like a ray of sunshine in my life." N.C. *"Your newsletters are great. I don't want to miss an issue." Wisconsin*	*"Your new format is great. I just love it and don't want to miss anything." Alberta, Canada* *"Your newsletter is very informative." Florida*

Subscribe today to this unique and timely newsletter!

() **1-year** subscription: **$23.00 In Canada $31.00 U.S.**

() **2-year** subscription: **$40.00 In Canada $51.00 U.S.**

() **3-year** subscription: **$46.00 In Canada $62.00 U.S.**

(3 yr best value. Get one year free with three!)

See order sheet on page 91.

Certified Reboundologist Workshop

The Ultimate Workshop for the Ultimate Exercise

3 Exciting Action-Filled Days

Creative sessions of rebounding incorporated with dynamic lectures, visual aids, videos, and group experiences are complimented with basic nutrition, spiritual, and mind-body connection information.

Linda will teach you how to successfully:

- Get the most from your rebounding experiences.
- Demonstrate proper use of the rebounder.
- Design individual rebounding programs.
- Motivate others to take charge of their health.
- Effectively advertise and develop a business.

Lectures and discussions include an in-depth study of the mechanics of rebounding and lymphatics in relation to many specific conditions, with emphasis on group study.

Daily rebound sessions, plus creative instructions for rebounding with seniors, children, weight loss, sports training, aerobics, vision, therapy, and much more.

Experience Rebounding! As you learn how this fascinating exercise flushes lymph, strengthens and oxygenates all cells, energizes, lifts spirits, and allows the body to heal, you will see many ways to incorporate rebound exercise into your personal healthy lifestyle and your health profession. Rebounding enhances and compliments all other therapeutic modalities.	**Early registration: $295.** (Paid up to 3 weeks prior to workshop) **Regular Tuition: $320.** For upcoming dates, full brochure, agenda, and registration information, contact: **Linda Brooks** **503 E. St. Clair St.** **Eaton, Ohio** **877-299-9547** **937-456-9633** **reboundvy@aol.com** **www.2rebound.com**

Product Order Sheet

Products	Quantity	Price	Total
____________________	______	____	____
____________________	______	____	____
____________________	______	____	____
____________________	______	____	____
____________________	______	____	____
____________________	______	____	____
____________________	______	____	____
____________________	______	____	____
____________________	______	____	____
____________________	______	____	____
			____

Product total	____
Shipping	____
O. res. 7.5% S.T.	____
Total	____

Shipping on books and videos: 10% of product total. Free shipping on $50 up and newsletter.

Mail or phone orders:
Visa, MC, Discover
Card # and exp date, check or money order.

Linda Brooks
503 E. St. Clair St.
Eaton, Ohio 45320
877-299-9547
937-456-9633
reboundvy@aol.com
www.2rebound.com

Product Order Sheet

Products	Quantity	Price	Total
______________________	______	____	____
______________________	______	____	____
______________________	______	____	____
______________________	______	____	____
______________________	______	____	____
______________________	______	____	____
______________________	______	____	____
______________________	______	____	____
______________________	______	____	____
______________________	______	____	____
			____
	Product total		____
	Shipping		____
	O. res. 7.5% S.T.		____
	Total		____

Mail or phone orders:
Visa, MC, Discover
Card # and exp date, check or money order.

Linda Brooks
503 E. St. Clair St.
Eaton, Ohio 45320
877-299-9547
937-456-9633
reboundvy@aol.com
www.2rebound.com

Shipping on books and videos: 10% of product total. Free shipping on $50 up and newsletter.

"You can *allow* yourself to become whole. You're never too old or too sick to dream and never too old or too sick to make dreams come true — *unless* you believe you are."

~~~Bob Trowbridge, *The Hidden Meaning of Illness*
~~~